INTUITIVE EATING 101

YOU WILL NEVER DIET AGAIN

ANGELA GLASER

Made with ♥ on the Notion Press Platform
www.notionpress.com

Contents

1

Intuitive Eating

Mindful eating, intuitive eating, and conscious eating are all terms used to describe a way of eating that uses internal cues about hunger, appetite and fullness to guide our relationship with food. Being attuned to and able to listen to our body allows us to know what and when we need to eat. The focus is on learning to eat in a conscious way that helps our body to feel and function well. Dieting, restricting, counting calories or fat grams and focusing on weight are NOT components of mindful eating. Mindful eaters eat when they are hungry and stop when they are satisfied. They eat the foods that they are hungry for. There is no list of "good" and "bad" foods.

Imagine if you had all the money you've ever spent on diet programs, what could you buy? Diamond earrings, a gold watch, a new car, a summer home? There is no doubt that those diets worked for you... short-term. But what happened after you went off the diet? More than likely, those pounds lost returned with an extra couple bonus pounds. Most diets will work because at the end of the day, when you cut your caloric intake, you will lose weight. But most people regain the weight lost because they have failed to make lifelong behavior changes. It is easier to follow a set of rules or pre-planned menus and see immediate results than to address the habits that caused them to put the weight on in the first place. That is why after following their diet rules for a period of time, and maybe even reaching their goal weight, they eventually gain it back. There is usually a trigger that occurs, be it an emotional upset, a major life change or escalating work stress that causes the individual to turn to food for comfort.

Every individual is born with the natural instinct to know when they are hungry and need to eat and when they are satisfied enough to stop eating. Think of when your children were born. Whether you breast-fed or bottle-fed your babies, they would cry when they were hungry and push away when they were full. As well-meaning parents (myself included) we would say "no, she didn't eat enough; there's 3 more ounces of formula left in the bottle". And we would try to feed the baby more, and the baby would push away again. When that baby became a little older and sat in a high chair, we would spoon-feed her and try all sorts of games, flying the spoon of peas through the air to song in order to get her to eat more. And then when they were toddlers, running around the house playing and not wanting to sit to eat lunch, we would worry that they would go hungry. But in fact, our children were exhibiting what was innate to them... the ability to eat when hungry and stop when full. So what happens over the years when you become an adult? Why can't you exhibit this same ability?

Well, some people might be able to look back at their childhood and remember that they were encouraged to "clean their plate" if they wanted dessert, or to tidy up their room and they'll go for an ice cream treat. These tactics all went against what was natural. And as you got older, the natural ability to tune into your hunger and satiety cues were further destroyed by the multi-billion-dollar diet business and the media exposure of the newest fad diet, the latest diet book or celebrity promoting some diet gimmick.

Intuitive eating is characterized by eating based on physiological hunger and satiety cues rather than situational and emotional cues. So simply said, you eat when you are hungry and you stop when you are satisfied. You do not eat because of boredom, loneliness, sadness, happiness, stress and anxiety. You do not eat because you are at a free buffet, or because there are cookies on the conference room table. You do not eat mindlessly, munching on a bag of chips while watching television. You do not engage in "conditioned eating behaviors" such as plowing through a bucket of popcorn at the movies because "that's what you do at the movies... eat popcorn." You eat solely when your body's signals tell you that you are hungry and you stop when you are comfortably full.

Every overweight person struggling to lose weight has this intuitive eater buried within them. The problem is that you have been looking for that magic bullet that will get the weight off NOW. So you try one diet after another, only to be disappointed when you regain the weight. You end up with very little trust in yourself, your body and the food you choose. I want you to know that you are not the one who failed. It's the diets that have failed you! So how do you become an intuitive eater? How do you reclaim what you were born with that will help you lose weight without ever going on another diet?

NOTE

- **Intuitive eating is the idea that if you listen to yourself you will find balance.**You will eat in a way connected to you and what your real needs are. Each of us intuitively knows deep down what we need. This goes for food as well, and what we eat can be a reflection of our body's true desires. Do you ever crave something deeply without knowing why? This kind of craving doesn't necessary linger for it is not picked up by the mind and obsessed over. It is not a thought of what you would like to eat, what you deserve or want. Instead it is your body sending you clues of what it needs, a flash of a message. These can be easy to overlook if we are not accustomed to listening.
- **It can be very easy to think our body is sending us a message to eat cake.** But remember this is a thought being processed not an instinct. To listen to your instincts, to allow yourself to be guided in this way, start by asking yourself with an open mind what you need. It can be quick and easy, no thoughts, no overriding desires, just a ?uick response. Your body knows what it needs; it doesn't really want to be buried by the things we obsess about.
- **Give your body the chance to be heard before you start eating,** before you go shopping or have a snack. Be aware of your impulses and before you react, ask yourself what you need. For that moment it could simply be a glass of water. You will find by listening you can nourish your body in a whole new way. By feeding yourself this way you will find unhealthy desires falling away, because your body's needs are being fulfilled and because you are listening. It can be easy, by practicing this method before

you eat, before you make a meal. Open the fridge or cupboard and let yourself intuitively guide your choices. Listen and you will become a far healthier you.

2

Here are 3 ways to get you started

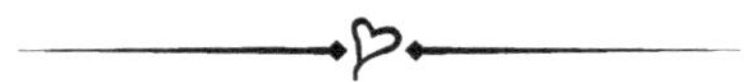

1. Reject the diet mentality! Make a decision to stop dieting! Throw out all the diet books that you have, all the pre-printed menus from the magazines that you cut out and all the diet rules and diet foods that you have tried. Make a commitment to yourself that you will no longer be influenced by the media or the next diet that comes to the market because if you let yourself be tempted again, it will prevent you from being free to rediscover intuitive eating.

2. Give yourself the unconditional permission to eat what you want when you want it. What happens when you deny yourself? When you crave a food but you don't "allow" yourself to eat it because it's not on your diet? At some point you give in to that craving and you typically overeat, or even binge on this forbidden food. By taking the conditions off the food and not labeling the food "bad", you will find that not only will you not overeat, but your true food preferences will be discovered.

3. Throw out the scale! Do you weigh yourself every morning or even several times per day? Does the number

on the scale influence your mood for the day? Most likely it does, even if you don't consciously realize it. Your weight fluctuates day-to- day and is a measure of more than just fat. It includes your bones, organs, muscle and substances such as water, food and waste that pass through your system. Begin to measure your success by other factors other than the scale such as improved blood work, blood pressure, mood, energy level and overall satisfaction with your progress toward becoming an intuitive eater.

3

Using Your Intuition to Eat

Most people are nutritionally unbalanced. The imbalance seems to come from an insufficiency of vitamins and minerals in the diet. The vitamins most likely to be out of balance are Vitamin D3, Vitamin B12 and Folic Acid. Other vitamins may be lacking as well, but most people are deficient in these. In addition to vitamins, most people are trace mineral deficient and some are potassium and magnesium deficient.

By correcting these deficiencies, which seem to alleviate most of the overeating symptoms, people seem to be more in tune with themselves and they can become more intuitive in their eating habits. By drinking more water, people notice they are not as hungry so they drink water first when they notice hunger signals. You begin to better interpret when you are hungry and when you are full. You are better able to decide what and how much to eat.

With intuitive eating, people don't worry so much about their body shape or how others see them. By focusing on how their body feels, they are better able to make intelligent food choice and improve their portion control. Their body size and shape naturally reformats to their ideal size.

People who become in tune with their bodies have much greater self-esteem, a higher stress reaction threshold so they are calmer, are more optimistic, are happier and have more positive emotions. They don't count calories or fat grams, drink disgusting diet potions, or starve themselves.

To start your process to become more intuitive in your eating style you need to throw out all of your diet books. They have rules that are imposed on you that throw you into a funk and make you feel guilty that yet another diet has failed. Stop the yo-yo effect. Diets only work while you are on them and most are impossible to sustain as part of a lifestyle choice.

If you think you are hungry, drink two glasses of water and wait a few minutes. If you are still hungry, for goodness sakes eat something. If you wait until you are over hungry, the food stuffing monster will appear and you will be out of control. It is actually best to eat five or six small meals or snacks in a day than to wait until you are over hungry.

Plan your mini-meals, so you know what you are going to be eating and you have all those good nutritious foods in the house. Intuit what your body would like to eat and incorporate as many colors and textures in your meals and snacks as possible. If you can do some raw, all the better. If your body needs something sweet, try making hot chocolate with almond milk and cocoa, sweetened with Stevia.

Let go of all your negative judgments around food. All of the things you should eat and all of the things you shouldn't are all surrounded by judgments lodged in your emotions. By creating a clear space around your food and your eating habits you become more intuitive as you develop your clarity.

Eat slowly and observe your body's signals. How does your food taste? Are you comfortably full yet? Don't be afraid to cover your food and refrigerate it until the next time you eat. It is not necessary to eat all the food on your plate. If you notice you are still hungry, by all means eat something else.

Be satisfied. The pleasure of eating delicious food in comfortable surroundings goes a long way to satisfy our hunger and our emotions around food. By eating in this way, you discover it takes much less food to bring you to a place of satisfaction.

If you're bummed out, recognize and deal with your emotions without eating. Notice that you are feeling down and recognize you are not in danger of exploding or other imminent disaster. You are feeling down at the moment but you will feel better. Food is to nourish your body, not to stuff into yourself for comfort. Do what you can to change the habit of using food for comfort.

Change the rules around food. Recognize when you are hungry and eat then. Do not eat when you are not. Any other excuse to eat is just that, an excuse. Have some character and some discipline around food. If you crave a carton of Chocolate Brownie Overload Ice Cream, make yourself a cup of hot chocolate with almond milk and Stevia. Make an agreement with yourself to break your food addictions. You will feel better for it and you can be more in control of what goes into your mouth.

No matter what you think you look like, respect yourself and love yourself no matter what your judgments are. The most critical eye in the world is yours. No one can be more self-critical than you and pick you apart like you can. Change your habit of your constant criti?uing and let yourself be who you really are. If all your relatives are round, you may have to be satisfied that you are round. You are not a horrible person if you have a muffin waist or a double chin.

Put on some walking shoes and go for a walk. If all you can manage right now is going to the end of the block and back, then you have done the best you can. Celebrate your achievements and look forward to walking around the block. By being in tune with yourself, you can progress at your own pace. Noticing how you feel and what progress you are making is a positive step.

Know that you are the only person that can restore your health and your waistline by making healthier food choices. Choose tasty, nutritious food that you feel good eating. Know that as you eat better you will feel better. As you feel better, you will want to feel even better. You will be encouraged by your progress and you will let your intuition guide you as you walk this new road of empowerment.

4

You Will Never Diet Again

Now that you've made the decision to stop dieting and want to become a normal or intuitive eater, you'll have to learn how to trust yourself around food. I'm talking about all those old tempting goodies that you used to avoid, play silly head games with or fear having in the house; the cookies, the lasagna, the cakes and pies, the breads, the chocolate, all those wonderful fattening tempties calling your name. Imagine all the yummies surrounding you; on your counter, in the cookie jar, stuffed in the pantry, the freezer, lined up in the cabinets, on shelves, in drawers, in your pocketbook, everywhere. No more hiding. No more running away. No more silly food games. No more guilt.

As a dieter, you've learned to think like a fat person and as long as you're thinking fat, you can never take steps that will make you thin. You're going to have to overhaul your thinking and clean it up in order for you to succeed at the task of listening to and rebuilding trust with your body. Making the commitment to change your relationship with food and your body is no small feat. You can be assured that there will be plenty of bumps along the way.

You'll have to retrain your brain how to think. Since our brains work on the basis of making pictures, it's not effective to use negative statements or words that will automatically be rejected by your subconscious mind. Because in order to make an image of the command, your brain would first have to picture you doing the things you don't want to do. For example, if I say, Don't eat the donut (as is a typical statement that a dieter might make), all your brain pictures is you eating the donut. Seeing that image is enough to trigger your memories of all the wonderful donuts you've enjoyed and before you know it, you're smack dab, knee deep, lost in memories, unable to decide if you want Krispy Kreme, Dunkin' Donuts, or mom's old fashioned home made apple cinnamon spice recipe. It's just that kind of brain tickle that puts you in a pickle, overstimulated enough to make you want to reach out and grab the next nearest donut or dozen to satisfy your desperate craving. So promise me. Don't say don't. Let's add that to the list.

5

Intuitive Eating For Natural Weight Loss

The human body is a miracle. It is built to take the best care of itself, if you let it. Eating is one of those things. If you learn how to listen to your body for cues of hunger and satiety, you will develop a healthier relationship with food. It might even be how to lose weight fast naturally; some people have lost tens of pounds just by following their inner signals.

Nowadays there is food available all the time, and many of us just don't know how it feels to be hungry. If we snack all the time, we don't get familiar with the feeling of hunger, nor the feeling of satiety. Here you can find four ways to learn to listen to your body more effectively.

How to start intuitive eating? The first thing to do is to learn how it feels to be hungry. This is the basis of the whole idea, so don't miss this one! The easiest way to start learning this is to create an eating routine. Eat three times a day, always at the same time. Do not eat in between meals. Soon your body will learn to follow this timetable and you will notice getting hungry before meal time. How does it feel to be hungry? How can you recognize being hungry?

The next step is to learn how it feels to have eaten enough. Do not limit your calorie intake during this period. Eat enough on each meal, but eat slowly. It takes about 10 minutes for the brain to realize that you have eaten something. Eat slowly and listen to your body. Stop eating when you feel satisfied and full, even if there is still food left. Explore the feeling of being satiated. Also, start assessing how much food it takes for you to feel full. It is usually less than you think.

Don't skip meals. Skipping meals will push you towards binge eating and snacking. Have proper meals throughout the day. Also, don't eat in front of the computer or the TV or read while eating. Concentrate on your food and on your body's signals. It is too easy to lose track of your inner feelings if you do other things while eating.

Eat enough. Don't be too strict on yourself. Limiting your diet too much and having these "eating rules" instead of listening to your internal cues can push you towards breaking the rules and binge eating. When you put intuitive eating into practice, you are free to eat anything your body desires. This food regime is not about forgetting healthy eating though. Listen to what your body wants you to eat, and to the internal cues of hunger and fullness.

For any weight loss approach to work, you have to be in the right frame of mind. Intuitive eating is not about abandoning your common sense, throwing caution to the wind and eating everything in sight. It doesn't give you license to eat poorly. (Your body actually prefers nutritious food.) It's about finding your personal happy healthy balance.

It's an approach that advocates being in tune with your hunger, sensible eating and allowing your body occasional indulgences without guilt. It's about freeing yourself from the food anxiety that is so prevalent in our society.

To be successful re?uires that you really learn about yourself and your eating habits and that you learn to be keenly aware of the situations that present big challenges for you and develop mechanisms for dealing with them.

Here are 7 healthy eating guidelines to help with your transition to an intuitive eating lifestyle. Although, I've committed them to memory, in the beginning, it's helpful to keep them posted where you can refer to them often.

Remember, these are not meant to be another set of rigid rules, but rather guiding principles to support you in developing a happy, healthy relationship with yourself. And remember, this is an ongoing process of self discovery, not a ?uick fix.

7 Guidelines for Intuitive Eating

1. Eat when you are physically hungry.
2. Eat sitting down in a calm environment.
3. Eat without distractions such as radio, television, newspapers, books, intense or anxiety provoking conversations or music.
4. Eat what your body wants. (Your body, not your spoiled inner child!)
5. Eat with the intention of being in full view of others.
6. Eat with enjoyment, gusto and pleasure.
7. Stop when you are full.

By committing to adopt and implement these guidelines, you will find yourself firmly planted on the path to anxiety free eating and weight loss, something wished everyone caught on the diet treadmill could discover.

6

Quick Ways Intuitive Eating Will Help You Lose Weight

There is a reason no current diet fads are sweeping the nation. It's because all that deprivation, starvation, and struggle don't work and haven't worked during the 100 year history of dieting. Look around at the people in your everyday life and it's obvious that all that dieting hasn't worked.

Instead, intuitive eating is an easy, graceful, natural approach to food. All we have to do is relearn a few simple things:

1. You have a brain in your belly. The medical community calls it the enteric system and it will guide you to the perfect foods, in the perfect amounts for your body to be its ideal weight. All you have to do is practice following the guidance it is constantly giving you.

2. Food is a wonderful, sensual part of life. Slowing down to really taste and enjoy your food will not only give you a delightful experience while you eat, it will also help you eat much less. As you practice mindful eating, you will find yourself enjoying food more and eating less.

3. Treat yourself well. You only get this one body and it is a wonder of creation. You deserve fresh air. You deserve wholesome, whole foods. Deprivation and struggle don't create a joyful life or a healthy body. Give your body the delights of delicious, unprocessed foods and playful movement as a way of taking loving care of yourself.

As you incorporate these new, entirely natural behaviors into your life, you will find you lose weight without having to make a great effort. Your body was born to be healthy and fit. You are naturally wired to be a normal weight. Honoring and listening to the natural wisdom of your body are skills that can be relearned. Intuitive eating is a powerful tool that will return you to your personal ideal weight with ease and grace.

If you're looking for a real, long-term solution to ending the battle with your weight, intuitive eating may just be the answer you've been seeking.

7

How to Listen to Your Hunger Cues

Intuitive eating is something that you can do for the rest of your life. Why? Because it is not a diet and it is not restrictive!

Diets bring you into a place of self restriction using "will power" (which is not real by the way). Once you reach your goal (or when you just cannot do it anymore) you give in. Your eating patterns resume to what they were before or worse.

Learning how to eat intuitively is especially helpful for those who suffer from emotional overeating and binge eating tendencies.

When it comes to emotional eating and binge eating; hunger cues become nonexistent. The line between emotional hunger and physical hunger is so blurred that there is no longer a distinction.

So how do you learn to eat intuitively?

Answer: Listen to Your Hunger Cues.

This is not when your mind says that you need a chocolate bar now! It's when your body physically tells you are in need of nutrition. This may come as a hallow feeling in your stomach or an actual "growl".

The first step in listening to your hunger cues is to make the distinction between emotional hunger and physical hunger.

You may want to begin keeping a journal to help you make that distinction. Write down what emotion you are feeling when you want to eat.

If you want something to eat because you're stressed or frustrated; ask yourself what would relieve that emotion instead of stuffing it away with food. You may want to take a walk to clear your mind and address the situation that is causing you to feel that way.

Numbing emotions with food is what got you where you are now... just give this a try and see what happens. You may still eat for emotional reasons in the beginning; but don't beat yourself up about it. Just acknowledge it and move on. If it is true physical hunger you are feeling; then eat whatever you want and stop when your stomach begins to feel comfortably full. In the beginning you may want a bowl of cookie dough. It's okay to do it; just make sure to stop when you're full. Eventually you will begin to want other foods and your diet will naturally become more nutritious.

A big problem for most people is knowing when to stop eating. We tend to eat because it tastes good and we don't want that sensation to end because it is pleasurable.

8

Tips For Creating an Enduring Habit of Intuitive Eating

When introduced to mindful eating, people often panic. "If there are no rules, I'll eat all day long." In the short run, some people do eat more, but mindful eating is not eating with abandon. Mindful eating is eating consciously, being aware of the present moment; being aware of hunger and fullness; being aware of your appetite and what you are really hungry for. Mindful or intuitive eating involves learning to be conscious of the difference between hunger and other eating cues such as painful emotions, boredom, or tiredness.

The Secret:

The secret to success with mindful or intuitive eating is this: You must remember or re-learn how to eat consciously--without shame, guilt, fear and with careful attention to your body and what it needs and wants. Doing this also re?uires learning what to do when what your body and mind need and want are not food. You must learn to listen respectfully to your body and learn to nourish your body and spirit without food when food is not what is called for.

The Essentials:

There are two essential components for creating an enduring habit of intuitive eating.

1. A Mindful Check-in Practice

The goal of mindful eating is to stop both obsessing about food/diet and stop going on automatic pilot with food/eating. In order to be successful, you will need to create a consistent method of checking in--staying connected with yourself and with what you are feeling and needing so that you can respond to these needs and desires and avoid emotional eating. You will need to find a practice that works for you and fits with your personality and your strengths. If the practice you choose doesn't suit you, you won't stick with it.

This may be something you do daily when you get up in the morning or before a meal or when you get home from work. The only requirements are that it be done consistently and that it is something that helps you focus inward, without distractions. It is often useful to have a few ways of doing mindful check-ins at various points in your day.

Examples of possible mindful check-ins: mindfulness meditation, journal writing or free writing, walking or running, prayer or contemplative time.

Often people start with writing. It might be useful to write about whatever is on your mind for fifteen minutes every morning. Especially in the beginning, it is helpful to keep an emotion/food log--noting how you are feeling and how hungry you are before you eat. The process of writing slows you down and forces you to think--to be mindful--of your eating.

2. A Support System

It is very important to have people (or a person) who support and encourage your belief system about not dieting. Your support system should honor your goals, celebrate your successes and help you stay accountable towards being the person you want to be. Your support system may help you to be consistent with your mindful practice. Your supporters know that you are not your weight or your clothing size. They are there for you when you doubt yourself or your path and when you hit roadblocks or find yourself in a place or with a feeling where you don't know what to do. They can help you figure out what to do when you know you are not hungry but feel like turning to food.

People create this support system in a variety of places. Your support may be available in friends you already have. Sometimes, however, the mindset of dieting is so entrenched in our families or social circle that it might be helpful to move outside your current life for support. A group, an online message board, or an intuitive eating class can be very helpful.

Disclaimer

Introduction

By using this book, you accept this disclaimer in full.

No advice

The book contains information. The information is not advice, and should not be treated as such.

If you think you may be suffering from any medical condition you should seek immediate medical attention. You should never delay seeking medical advice, disregard medical advice, or discontinue medical treatment because of information in the book.

No representations or warranties

To the maximum extent permitted by applicable law and subject to section below, we exclude all representations, warranties, undertakings and guarantees relating to the book.

Without prejudice to the generality of the foregoing paragraph, we do not represent, warrant, undertake or guarantee:

- that the information in the book is correct, accurate, complete or non-misleading;

- that the use of the guidance in the book will lead to any particular outcome or result.

Limitations and exclusions of liability

The limitations and exclusions of liability set out in this section and elsewhere in this disclaimer: are subject to section 6 below; and govern all liabilities arising under the disclaimer or in relation to the book, including liabilities arising in contract, in tort (including negligence) and for breach of statutory duty.

We will not be liable to you in respect of any losses arising out of any event or events beyond our reasonable control.

We will not be liable to you in respect of any business losses, including without limitation loss of or damage to profits, income, revenue, use, production, anticipated savings, business, contracts, commercial opportunities or goodwill.

We will not be liable to you in respect of any loss or corruption of any data, database or software.

We will not be liable to you in respect of any special, indirect or consequential loss or damage.

Exceptions

Nothing in this disclaimer shall: limit or exclude our liability for death or personal injury resulting from negligence; limit or exclude our liability for fraud or fraudulent misrepresentation; limit any of our liabilities in any way that is not permitted under applicable law; or exclude any of our liabilities that may not be excluded under applicable law.

Severability

If a section of this disclaimer is determined by any court or other competent authority to be unlawful and/ or unenforceable, the other sections of this disclaimer continue in effect.

If any unlawful and/or unenforceable section would be lawful or enforceable if part of it were deleted, that part will be deemed to be deleted, and the rest of the section will continue in effect.

Law and jurisdiction

This disclaimer will be governed by and construed in accordance with Swiss law, and any disputes relating to this disclaimer will be subject to the exclusive jurisdiction of the courts of Switzerland.

9 798888 838884

Printed by Libri Plureos GmbH in Hamburg, Germany